# Healthy Weight Loss for Kids
# and the Young at Heart

Healthy Weight Loss for Kids and the Young at Heart

Karen L. Aken

ISBN-13: 978-1518858666
ISBN-10: 151885866X

## Introduction

A healthy weight loss is only about a quarter of a pound to two pounds per week depending on your age and size. If you follow the advice in this journal you will reach a healthy weight for your age. Invite your parents or friends to join you. Challenge others to do some or all of the goals that I have created for you. Please try to follow all of these goals even if you think they are silly or weird. These goals are meant to improve your mind, body, and soul. Please consult your doctor before beginning this or any other exercise program.

# Day One

## Goals

- Drink 6-8 glasses of water* (no flavor added, just WATER)
- Walk **or** jog (anywhere, inside or out) **or** march in place for at least 5 minutes
- Shut off all electronics for 2 minutes, except for one that you will only use as a timer, go to a quiet space, set your timer, sit comfortably, close your eyes, take deep breaths and focus only on the air flowing into your nose, down into your lungs, and back out again, repeat until time is up.
- Something I am thankful for today:
- Notes: (Anything you would like to add, how you did, how your day was, etc.)

*Never drink 6-8 glasses of water all at once, this can be harmful to your health. Please drink your water at a slow pace throughout the day.

# Day Two

## Goals

- Drink 6-8 glasses of water (no flavor added, just WATER)
- Go for a walk, jog or march in place for at least 5 minutes
- For 2 minutes, go to a quiet space, sit comfortably, close your eyes, take deep breaths, focus only on the air flowing into your nose, down into your lungs, and back out again.
- **Stand on one leg and count to 10, stand on the other and count to 10\***
- Something I am thankful for today:
- Notes:

\*This will improve your balance and also works your stomach muscles aka your abs or core

# Day Three

## Goals

- Drink 6-8 glasses of water (no flavor added, just WATER)
- Go for a walk, jog or march in place for at least 5 minutes
- For 2 minutes, go to a quiet space, sit comfortably, close your eyes, take deep breaths, focus only on the air flowing into your nose, down into your lungs, and back out again.
- Stand on one leg and count to 10, then the other and count to 10
- **Do 10 Jumping Jacks***
- Something I am thankful for today:
- Notes:

*This is a cardiovascular exercise aka cardio. Cardiovascular exercise is any exercise that increases your heart rate. It makes your body stronger and healthier.

# Day Four

## Goals

- Drink 6-8 glasses of water (no flavor added, just WATER)
- Go for a walk, jog or march in place for at least 5 minutes
- For 2 minutes, go to a quiet space, sit comfortably, close your eyes, take deep breaths, focus only on the air flowing into your nose, down into your lungs, and back out again.
- Stand on one leg and count to 10, then the other and count to 10
- Do 10 Jumping Jacks (cardio)
- **Eat at least one whole piece of fruit (an apple, banana, orange, whatever your favorite fruit is)**
- Something I am thankful for today:
- Notes:

*Health Tip: Never go more than 4 hours without eating (unless you are sleeping). After 4 hours your body slows down it's metabolism because your body thinks it might starve. This also happens when you don't eat breakfast. A slow metabolism can make you gain weight.

# Day Five

## Goals

- Drink 6-8 glasses of water (no flavor added, just WATER)
- Go for a walk, jog or march in place for at least 5 minutes
- For 2 minutes, go to a quiet space, sit comfortably, close your eyes, take deep breaths, focus only on the air flowing into your nose, down into your lungs, and back out again.
- Stand on one leg and count to 10, then the other and count to 10
- Do 10 Jumping Jacks
- **Do 5 sit-ups or hula hoop for 15 seconds in one direction and 15 seconds in the other direction (you don't have to have a hula hoop, you can pretend that you are using one).\***
- Eat at least one whole piece of fruit
- Something I am thankful for today:
- Notes:

\*These exercises improve your stomach muscles. They also improve your balance and help your entire body move better.

# Day Six

## Goals

- Drink 6-8 glasses of water (no flavor added, just WATER)
- Go for a walk, jog or march in place for at least 5 minutes
- For 2 minutes, go to a quiet space, sit comfortably, close your eyes, take deep breaths, focus only on the air flowing into your nose, down into your lungs, and back out again.
- Stand on one leg and count to 10, then the other and count to 10
- Do 10 Jumping Jacks
- Do 5 sit-ups or hula hoop for 15 seconds in one direction and 15 seconds in the other direction
- Eat at least one whole piece of fruit
- Something I am thankful for today:
- Notes:

*Health Tip: Let the grocery shopper in your home know that generic and store brands often contain more high fructose corn syrup (HFCS) than other brands. Eating or drinking products that contain HFCS is not good for your health.

# Day Seven

## Goals

- Drink 6-8 glasses of water (no flavor added, just WATER)
- Go for a walk, jog or march in place for at least 5 minutes
- For **3** minutes, go to a quiet space, sit comfortably, close your eyes, take deep breaths, focus only on the air flowing into your nose, down into your lungs, and back out again.*
- Stand on one leg and count to 10, then the other and count to 10
- Do 10 Jumping Jacks
- Do 5 sit-ups or hula hoop for 15 seconds in one direction and 15 seconds in the other direction
- Eat at least one whole piece of fruit
- Something I am thankful for today:
- Something I like about myself:
- Notes:

*Have you wondered why I keep making you do this yet? You have been practicing meditation. This is one of the best and easiest ways to improve your overall health.

# Day Eight

## Goals

- Drink 6-8 glasses of water (no flavor added, just WATER)
- Go for a walk, jog or march in place for at least **7** minutes
- For 3 minutes, go to a quiet space, sit comfortably, close your eyes, take deep breaths, focus only on the air flowing into your nose, down into your lungs, and back out again.
- Stand on one leg and count to 10, then the other and count to 10
- Do 10 Jumping Jacks
- Do 5 sit-ups or hula hoop for 15 seconds in one direction and 15 seconds in the other direction
- Eat at least one whole piece of fruit
- Something I am thankful for today:
- Something I like about myself:
- Notes:

*Health Tip: Singing burns calories (about 10 calories per song) and exercises your heart and your lungs. It can also cheer you up.

# Day Nine

## Goals

- Drink 6-8 glasses of water (no flavor added, just WATER)
- Go for a walk, jog or march in place for at least 7 minutes
- For 3 minutes, go to a quiet space, sit comfortably, close your eyes, take deep breaths, focus only on the air flowing into your nose, down into your lungs, and back out again.
- Stand on one leg and count to **15**, then the other and count to **15**
- Do 10 Jumping Jacks
- Do 5 sit-ups or hula hoop for 15 seconds in one direction and 15 seconds in the other direction
- Eat at least one whole piece of fruit
- Something I am thankful for today:
- Something I like about myself:
- Notes:

*Health Tip: Let the cook in your family know that ground turkey is healthier than ground beef. Ground turkey has less saturated fats. Saturated fats are not good for your heart or your body.

# Day Ten

## Goals

- Drink 6-8 glasses of water (no flavor added, just WATER)
- Go for a walk, jog or march in place for at least 7 minutes
- For 3 minutes, go to a quiet space, sit comfortably, close your eyes, take deep breaths, focus only on the air flowing into your nose, down into your lungs, and back out again.
- Stand on one leg and count to 15, then the other and count to 15
- Do 15 Jumping Jacks
- Do 5 sit-ups or hula hoop for 15 seconds in one direction and 15 seconds in the other direction
- Eat at least one whole piece of fruit
- Something I am thankful for today:
- Something I like about myself:
- Notes:

*Health Tip: Gatorade and other sports drinks are just as unhealthy as soda. It is not a good idea to drink sports drinks unless you are playing a sport, running, or exercising for long periods of time (over 60 minutes) or spending a lot of time outside when it's hot.

# Day Eleven

## Goals

- Drink 6-8 glasses of water (no flavor added, just WATER)
- Go for a walk, jog or march in place for at least 7 minutes
- For 3 minutes, go to a quiet space, sit comfortably, close your eyes, take deep breaths, focus only on the air flowing into your nose, down into your lungs, and back out again.
- Stand on one leg and count to 15, then the other and count to 15
- Do 15 Jumping Jacks
- Do 5 sit-ups or hula hoop for 15 seconds in one direction and 15 seconds in the other direction
- Eat at least one whole piece of fruit
- **Eat at least one 1/2 cup of vegetables (peas, green beans, carrots, whatever your favorite vegetable is)**
- Something I am thankful for today:
- Something I like about myself:
- Notes:

*Health Tip: Let the cook in your family know that frozen fruits and vegetables are healthier than canned because they contain less salt and sugar. They also cost less.

# Day Twelve

## Goals

- Drink 6-8 glasses of water (no flavor added, just WATER)
- Go for a walk, jog or march in place for at least 7 minutes
- Shut off all electronics for 3 minutes, go to a quiet space, sit comfortably, close your eyes, take deep breaths, focus only on the air flowing into your nose, down into your lungs, and back out again.
- Stand on one leg and count to 15, then the other and count to 15
- Do 15 Jumping Jacks
- Do 10 sit-ups or hula hoop for 20 seconds in one direction and 20 seconds in the other direction
- Eat at least one whole piece of fruit
- Eat at least one 1/2 cup of vegetables
- Something I am thankful for today:
- Something I like about myself:
- Notes:

*Health Tip: Turning off all of your electronic devices at least 30 minutes before you go to bed and dimming the lights will help you fall asleep faster.

# Day Thirteen

## Goals

- Drink 6-8 glasses of water (no flavor added, just WATER)
- Go for a walk, jog or march in place for at least 7 minutes
- Shut off all electronics for 3 minutes, go to a quiet space, sit comfortably, close your eyes, take deep breaths, focus only on the air flowing into your nose, down into your lungs, and back out again.
- Stand on one leg and count to 15, then the other and count to 15
- Do 15 Jumping Jacks
- Do 10 sit-ups or hula hoop for 20 seconds in one direction and 20 seconds in the other direction
- Eat at least one whole piece of fruit
- Eat at least one 1/2 cup of vegetables
- Something I am thankful for today:
- Something I like about myself:
- Notes:

*Health Tip: Fat is not always bad for you. Your body needs fat for things like energy and to keep you warm. Vegetables, nuts, seeds, and fish contain healthy fats. Cookies, cake, and chips do not.

# Day Fourteen

## Goals

- Drink 6-8 glasses of water (no flavor added, just WATER)
- Go for a walk, jog or march in place for at least 7 minutes
- Shut off all electronics for **4** minutes, go to a quiet space, sit comfortably, close your eyes, take deep breaths, focus only on the air flowing into your nose, down into your lungs, and back out again.
- Stand on one leg and count to 15, then the other and count to 15
- Do 15 Jumping Jacks
- Do 10 sit-ups or hula hoop for 20 seconds in one direction and 20 seconds in the other direction
- Eat at least one whole piece of fruit
- Eat at least one 1/2 cup of vegetables
- Something I am thankful for today:
- Something I like about myself:
- **Something nice I did for someone else today:**

- Notes:

*Health Tip: Hoola hooping is a great way to work your stomach muscles. It also burns about 5 calories per minute.

# Day Fifteen

## Goals

- Drink 6-8 glasses of water (no flavor added, just WATER)
- Go for a walk, jog or march in place for at least **9** minutes
- Shut off all electronics for 4 minutes, go to a quiet space, sit comfortably, close your eyes, take deep breaths, focus only on the air flowing into your nose, down into your lungs, and back out again.
- Stand on one leg and count to 15, then the other and count to 15
- Do 15 Jumping Jacks
- Do 10 sit-ups or hula hoop for 20 seconds in one direction and 20 seconds in the other direction
- Eat at least one whole piece of fruit
- Eat at least one 1/2 cup of vegetables
- Something I am thankful for today:
- Something I like about myself:
- Something nice I did for someone else today:

- Notes:

*Health Tip: Yellow vegetables are good for your skin, teeth, and bones.

# Day Sixteen

## Goals

- Drink 6-8 glasses of water (no flavor added, just WATER)
- Go for a walk, jog or march in place for at least 9 minutes
- Shut off all electronics for 4 minutes, go to a quiet space, sit comfortably, close your eyes, take deep breaths, focus only on the air flowing into your nose, down into your lungs, and back out again.
- Stand on one leg and count to **20**, then the other and count to **20**
- Do 15 Jumping Jacks
- Do 10 sit-ups or hula hoop for 20 seconds in one direction and 20 seconds in the other direction
- Eat at least one whole piece of fruit
- Eat at least one 1/2 cup of vegetables
- Something I am thankful for today:
- Something I like about myself:
- Something nice I did for someone else today:

- Notes:

*Health Tip: Laughing is good for your mind, your body, and your heart.

# Day Seventeen

## Goals

- Drink 6-8 glasses of water (no flavor added, just WATER)
- Go for a walk, jog or march in place for at least 9 minutes
- Shut off all electronics for 4 minutes, go to a quiet space, sit comfortably, close your eyes, take deep breaths, focus only on the air flowing into your nose, down into your lungs, and back out again.
- Stand on one leg and count to 20, then the other and count to 20
- Do **20** Jumping Jacks
- Do 10 sit-ups or hula hoop for 20 seconds in one direction and 20 seconds in the other direction
- Eat at least one whole piece of fruit
- Eat at least one 1/2 cup of vegetables
- Something I am thankful for today:
- Something I like about myself:
- Something nice I did for someone else today:

- Notes:

*Health Tip: Red fruits and vegetables are good for your heart.

# Day Eighteen

## Goals

- Drink 6-8 glasses of water (no flavor added, just WATER)
- Go for a walk, jog or march in place for at least 9 minutes
- Shut off all electronics for 4 minutes, go to a quiet space, sit comfortably, close your eyes, take deep breaths, focus only on the air flowing into your nose, down into your lungs, and back out again.
- Stand on one leg and count to 20, then the other and count to 20
- Do 20 Jumping Jacks
- Do 10 sit-ups or hula hoop for 20 seconds in one direction and 20 seconds in the other direction
- Eat at least **two** whole pieces of fruit
- Eat at least one 1/2 cup of vegetables
- Something I am thankful for today:
- Something I like about myself:
- Something nice I did for someone else today:

- Notes:

*Health tip: Going to bed at the same time and waking up at the same time every day is a simple way to improve your health.

# Day Nineteen

## Goals

- Drink 6-8 glasses of water (no flavor added, just WATER)
- Go for a walk, jog or march in place for at least 9 minutes
- Shut off all electronics for 4 minutes, go to a quiet space, sit comfortably, close your eyes, take deep breaths, focus only on the air flowing into your nose, down into your lungs, and back out again.
- Stand on one leg and count to 20, then the other and count to 20
- Do 20 Jumping Jacks
- Do **15** sit-ups or hula hoop for **25** seconds in one direction and **25** seconds in the other direction
- Eat at least two whole pieces of fruit
- Eat at least one 1/2 cup of vegetables
- Something I am thankful for today:
- Something I like about myself:
- Something nice I did for someone else today:

- Notes:

*Health Tip: Listening to music helps motivate you, improves your memory, and puts you in a good mood.

# Day Twenty

## Goals

- Drink 6-8 glasses of water (no flavor added, just WATER)
- Go for a walk, jog or march in place for at least 9 minutes
- Shut off all electronics for 4 minutes, go to a quiet space, sit comfortably, close your eyes, take deep breaths, focus only on the air flowing into your nose, down into your lungs, and back out again.
- Stand on one leg and count to 20, then the other and count to 20
- Do 20 Jumping Jacks
- Do 15 sit-ups or hula hoop for 25 seconds in one direction and 25 seconds in the other direction
- Eat at least two whole pieces of fruit
- Eat at least one 1/2 cup of vegetables
- Something I am thankful for today:
- Something I like about myself:
- Something nice I did for someone else today:

- Notes:

*Health Tip: Make a rule for yourself that if you are going to snack while watching TV, you only snack on fruits or vegetables.

# Day Twenty-One

## Goals

- Drink 6-8 glasses of water (no flavor added, just WATER)
- Go for a walk, jog or march in place for at least 9 minutes
- Shut off all electronics for **5** minutes, go to a quiet space, sit comfortably, close your eyes, take deep breaths, focus only on the air flowing into your nose, down into your lungs, and back out again.
- Stand on one leg and count to 20, then the other and count to 20
- Do 20 Jumping Jacks
- Do 15 sit-ups or hula hoop for 25 seconds in one direction and 25 seconds in the other direction
- **With your arms straight out from your sides, do arm circles 10 forward, 10 backward, big or small.**
- Eat at least two whole pieces of fruit
- Eat at least one 1/2 cup of vegetables
- **Choose your own goal: (example: quit drinking soda)**
- Something I am thankful for today:
- Something I like about myself:
- Something nice I did for someone else today:


- Notes:

\*Health Tip: Jumping rope improves coordination, makes your bones strong, and burns more calories than jogging.

# Day Twenty-Two

## Goals

- Drink 6-8 glasses of water (no flavor added, just WATER)
- Go for a walk, jog or march in place for at least 11 minutes
- Shut off all electronics for 5 minutes, go to a quiet space, sit comfortably, close your eyes, take deep breaths, focus only on the air flowing into your nose, down into your lungs, and back out again.
- Stand on one leg and count to 20, then the other and count to 20
- Do 20 Jumping Jacks
- Do 15 sit-ups or hula hoop for 25 seconds in one direction and 25 seconds in the other direction
- Do arm circles 10 forward, 10 backward, big or small.
- Eat at least two whole pieces of fruit
- Eat at least one 1/2 cup of vegetables
- My goal:
- Something I am thankful for today:
- Something I like about myself:
- Something nice I did for someone else today:

- Notes:


*Health Tip: Swinging on a swing burns 100 calories in 30 minutes.

# Day Twenty-Three

## Goals

- Drink 6-8 glasses of water (no flavor added, just WATER)
- Go for a walk, jog or march in place for at least 11 minutes
- Shut off all electronics for 5 minutes, go to a quiet space, sit comfortably, close your eyes, take deep breaths, focus only on the air flowing into your nose, down into your lungs, and back out again.
- Stand on one leg and count to **25**, then the other and count to **25**
- Do 20 Jumping Jacks
- Do 15 sit-ups or hula hoop for 25 seconds in one direction and 25 seconds in the other direction
- Do arm circles 10 forward, 10 backward, big or small.
- Eat at least two whole pieces of fruit
- Eat at least one 1/2 cup of vegetables
- My goal:
- Something I am thankful for today:
- Something I like about myself:
- Something nice I did for someone else today:

- Notes:


*Health Tip: Purple fuits and vegetables are good for your heart.

# Day Twenty-Four

## Goals

- Drink 6-8 glasses of water (no flavor added, just WATER)
- Go for a walk, jog or march in place for at least 11 minutes
- Shut off all electronics for 5 minutes, go to a quiet space, sit comfortably, close your eyes, take deep breaths, focus only on the air flowing into your nose, down into your lungs, and back out again.
- Stand on one leg and count to 25, then the other and count to 25*
- Do **25** Jumping Jacks
- Do 15 sit-ups or hula hoop for 25 seconds in one direction and 25 seconds in the other direction
- Do arm circles 10 forward, 10 backward, big or small.
- Eat at least two whole pieces of fruit
- Eat at least one 1/2 cup of vegetables
- My goal:
- Something I am thankful for today:
- Something I like about myself:
- Something nice I did for someone else today:

- Notes:

*Health Tip: To make standing on one leg harder, close your eyes.

# Day Twenty-Five

## Goals

- Drink 6-8 glasses of water (no flavor added, just WATER)
- Go for a walk, jog or march in place for at least 11 minutes
- Shut off all electronics for 5 minutes, go to a quiet space, sit comfortably, close your eyes, take deep breaths, focus only on the air flowing into your nose, down into your lungs, and back out again.
- Stand on one leg and count to 25, then the other and count to 25
- Do 25 Jumping Jacks
- Do 15 sit-ups or hula hoop for 25 seconds in one direction and 25 seconds in the other direction
- Do arm circles 10 forward, 10 backward, big or small.
- Eat at least two whole pieces of fruit
- Eat at least **one cup** of vegetables
- My goal:
- Something I am thankful for today:
- Something I like about myself:
- Something nice I did for someone else today:

- Notes:

*Health Tip: Green fruits and vegetables are good for your eyes, bones, and teeth.

# Day Twenty-Six

## Goals

- Drink 6-8 glasses of water (no flavor added, just WATER)
- Go for a walk, jog or march in place for at least 11 minutes
- Shut off all electronics for 5 minutes, go to a quiet space, sit comfortably, close your eyes, take deep breaths, focus only on the air flowing into your nose, down into your lungs, and back out again.
- Stand on one leg and count to 25, then the other and count to 25
- Do 25 Jumping Jacks
- Do **20** sit-ups or hula hoop for **30** seconds in one direction and **30** seconds in the other direction
- Do arm circles 10 forward, 10 backward, big or small.
- Eat at least two whole pieces of fruit
- Eat at least one cup of vegetables
- My goal:
- Something I am thankful for today:
- Something I like about myself:
- Something nice I did for someone else today:

- Notes:

*Health Tip: Eat breakfast within 2 hours of waking up to give your body and your brain energy. The sooner the better!

# Day Twenty-Seven

## Goals

- Drink 6-8 glasses of water (no flavor added, just WATER)
- Go for a walk, jog or march in place for at least 11 minutes
- Shut off all electronics for 5 minutes, go to a quiet space, sit comfortably, close your eyes, take deep breaths, focus only on the air flowing into your nose, down into your lungs, and back out again.
- Stand on one leg and count to 25, then the other and count to 25
- Do 25 Jumping Jacks
- Do 20 sit-ups or hula hoop for 30 seconds in one direction and 30 seconds in the other direction
- Do arm circles 10 forward, 10 backward, big or small.
- Eat at least two whole pieces of fruit
- Eat at least one cup of vegetables
- My goal:
- Something I am thankful for today:
- Something I like about myself:
- Something nice I did for someone else today:

- Notes:

*Health Tip: Orange fruits and vegetables are good for your eyes and your skin. They also strengthen your immunity.

# Day Twenty-Eight

## Goals

- Drink 6-8 glasses of water (no flavor added, just WATER)
- Go for a walk, jog or march in place for at least 11 minutes
- Shut off all electronics for 6 minutes, go to a quiet space, sit comfortably, close your eyes, take deep breaths, focus only on the air flowing into your nose, down into your lungs, and back out again.
- Stand on one leg and count to 25, then the other and count to 25
- Do 25 Jumping Jacks
- Do 20 sit-ups or hula hoop for 30 seconds in one direction and 30 seconds in the other direction
- Do arm circles 15 forward, 15 backward, big or small.
- Eat at least two whole pieces of fruit
- Eat at least one cup of vegetables
- My goal:
- Something I am thankful for today:
- Something I like about myself:
- Something nice I did for someone else today:

- Notes:

*Health Tip: Standing burns more calories than sitting.

# Day Twenty-Nine

## Goals

- Drink 6-8 glasses of water (no flavor added, just WATER)
- Go for a walk, jog or march in place for at least **13** minutes
- Shut off all electronics for 6 minutes, go to a quiet space, sit comfortably, close your eyes, take deep breaths, focus only on the air flowing into your nose, down into your lungs, and back out again.
- Stand on one leg and count to 25, then the other and count to 25
- Do 25 Jumping Jacks
- Do 20 sit-ups or hula hoop for 30 seconds in one direction and 30 seconds in the other direction
- Do arm circles 15 forward, 15 backward, big or small.
- Eat at least two whole pieces of fruit
- Eat at least one cup of vegetables
- My goal:
- Something I am thankful for today:
- Something I like about myself:
- Something nice I did for someone else today:

- Notes:


*Health Tip: Swimming is good for your heart and your lungs.

# Day Thirty

## Goals

- Drink 6-8 glasses of water (no flavor added, just WATER)
- Go for a walk, jog or march in place for at least 13 minutes
- Shut off all electronics for 6 minutes, go to a quiet space, sit comfortably, close your eyes, take deep breaths, focus only on the air flowing into your nose, down into your lungs, and back out again.
- Stand on one leg and count to **30**, then the other and count to **30**
- Do 25 Jumping Jacks
- Do 20 sit-ups or hula hoop for 30 seconds in one direction and 30 seconds in the other direction
- Do arm circles 15 forward, 15 backward, big or small.
- Eat at least two whole pieces of fruit
- Eat at least one cup of vegetables
- My goal:
- Something I am thankful for today:
- Something I like about myself:
- Something nice I did for someone else today:

- Notes:


*Health Tip: Smile! It makes you happy and relaxes your body.

# Day Thirty-One

## Goals

- Drink 6-8 glasses of water (no flavor added, just WATER)
- Go for a walk, jog or march in place for at least 13 minutes
- Shut off all electronics for 6 minutes, go to a quiet space, sit comfortably, close your eyes, take deep breaths, focus only on the air flowing into your nose, down into your lungs, and back out again.
- Stand on one leg and count to 30, then the other and count to 30
- Do **30** Jumping Jacks
- Do 20 sit-ups or hula hoop for 30 seconds in one direction and 30 seconds in the other direction
- Do arm circles 15 forward, 15 backward, big or small.
- Eat at least two whole pieces of fruit
- Eat at least one cup of vegetables
- My goal:
- Something I am thankful for today:
- Something I like about myself:
- Something nice I did for someone else today:

- Notes:


*Health Tip: White fruits and vegetables are good for your bones.

# Day Thirty-Two

## Goals

- Drink 6-8 glasses of water (no flavor added, just WATER)
- Go for a walk, jog or march in place for at least 13 minutes
- Shut off all electronics for 6 minutes, go to a quiet space, sit comfortably, close your eyes, take deep breaths, focus only on the air flowing into your nose, down into your lungs, and back out again.
- Stand on one leg and count to 30, then the other and count to 30
- Do 30 Jumping Jacks
- Do 20 sit-ups or hula hoop for 30 seconds in one direction and 30 seconds in the other direction
- Do arm circles 15 forward, 15 backward, big or small.
- Eat at least two whole pieces of fruit
- Eat at least **one and a half cups** of vegetables
- My goal:
- Something I am thankful for today:
- Something I like about myself:
- Something nice I did for someone else today:

- Notes:

*Health Tip: Forgiving others is good for your heart.

# Day Thirty-Three

## Goals

- Drink 6-8 glasses of water (no flavor added, just WATER)
- Go for a walk, jog or march in place for at least 13 minutes
- Shut off all electronics for 6 minutes, go to a quiet space, sit comfortably, close your eyes, take deep breaths, focus only on the air flowing into your nose, down into your lungs, and back out again.
- Stand on one leg and count to 30, then the other and count to 30
- Do 30 Jumping Jacks
- Do **25** sit-ups or hula hoop for **35** seconds in one direction and **35** seconds in the other direction
- Do arm circles 15 forward, 15 backward, big or small.
- Eat at least two whole pieces of fruit
- Eat at least one and a half cups of vegetables
- My goal:
- Something I am thankful for today:
- Something I like about myself:
- Something nice I did for someone else today:

- Notes:

*Health Tip: Try balancing on one leg and then the other while brushing your teeth.

# Day Thirty-Four

## Goals

- Drink 6-8 glasses of water (no flavor added, just WATER)
- Go for a walk, jog or march in place for at least 13 minutes
- Shut off all electronics for 6 minutes, go to a quiet space, sit comfortably, close your eyes, take deep breaths, focus only on the air flowing into your nose, down into your lungs, and back out again.
- Stand on one leg and count to 30, then the other and count to 30
- Do 30 Jumping Jacks
- Do 25 sit-ups or hula hoop for 35 seconds in one direction and 35 seconds in the other direction
- Do arm circles 15 forward, 15 backward, big or small.
- Eat at least two whole pieces of fruit
- Eat at least one and a half cups of vegetables
- My goal:
- Something I am thankful for today:
- Something I like about myself:
- Something nice I did for someone else today:

- Notes:

*Health Tip: Even your eyes can be at risk for sunburn. Wearing sunglasses can prevent eye problems now and later on in life.

# Day Thirty-Five

## Goals

- Drink 6-8 glasses of water (no flavor added, just WATER)
- Go for a walk, jog or march in place for at least 13 minutes
- Shut off all electronics for **7** minutes, go to a quiet space, sit comfortably, close your eyes, take deep breaths, focus only on the air flowing into your nose, down into your lungs, and back out again.
- Stand on one leg and count to 30, then the other and count to 30
- Do 30 Jumping Jacks
- Do 25 sit-ups or hula hoop for 35 seconds in one direction and 35 seconds in the other direction
- Do arm circles **20** forward, **20** backward, big or small.
- Eat at least two whole pieces of fruit
- Eat at least one and a half cups of vegetables
- My goal: **(keep this goal or change it)**
- **Time for another goal: (example: train for a 5k)**
- Something I am thankful for today:
- Something I like about myself:
- Something nice I did for someone else today:

- Notes:

# Day Thirty-Six

## Goals

- Drink 6-8 glasses of water (no flavor added, just WATER)
- Go for a walk, jog or march in place for at least **15** minutes
- Shut off all electronics for 7 minutes, go to a quiet space, sit comfortably, close your eyes, take deep breaths, focus only on the air flowing into your nose, down into your lungs, and back out again.
- Stand on one leg and count to 30, then the other and count to 30
- Do 30 Jumping Jacks
- Do 25 sit-ups or hula hoop for 35 seconds in one direction and 35 seconds in the other direction
- Do arm circles 20 forward, 20 backward, big or small.
- Eat at least two whole pieces of fruit
- Eat at least one and a half cups of vegetables
- 1st goal:
- 2nd goal:
- Something I am thankful for today:
- Something I like about myself:
- Something nice I did for someone else today:

- Notes:

# Day Thirty-Seven

## Goals

- Drink 6-8 glasses of water (no flavor added, just WATER)
- Go for a walk, jog or march in place for at least 15 minutes
- Shut off all electronics for 7 minutes, go to a quiet space, sit comfortably, close your eyes, take deep breaths, focus only on the air flowing into your nose, down into your lungs, and back out again.
- **Hop** on one leg and count to **10**, then the other and count to **10**
- Do 30 Jumping Jacks
- Do 25 sit-ups or hula hoop for 35 seconds in one direction and 35 seconds in the other direction
- Do arm circles 20 forward, 20 backward, big or small.
- Eat at least two whole pieces of fruit
- Eat at least one and a half cups of vegetables
- 1st goal:
- 2nd goal:
- Something I am thankful for today:
- Something I like about myself:
- Something nice I did for someone else today:

- Notes:

# Day Thirty-Eight

## Goals

- Drink 6-8 glasses of water (no flavor added, just WATER)
- Go for a walk, jog or march in place for at least 15 minutes
- Shut off all electronics for 7 minutes, go to a quiet space, sit comfortably, close your eyes, take deep breaths, focus only on the air flowing into your nose, down into your lungs, and back out again.
- Hop on one leg and count to 10, then the other and count to 10
- Do **35** Jumping Jacks
- Do 25 sit-ups or hula hoop for 35 seconds in one direction and 35 seconds in the other direction
- Do arm circles 20 forward, 20 backward, big or small.
- Eat at least two whole pieces of fruit
- Eat at least one and a half cups of vegetables
- 1st goal:
- 2nd goal:
- Something I am thankful for today:
- Something I like about myself:
- Something nice I did for someone else today:

- Notes:

# Day Thirty-Nine

## Goals

- Drink 6-8 glasses of water (no flavor added, just WATER)
- Go for a walk, jog or march in place for at least 15 minutes
- Shut off all electronics for 7 minutes, go to a quiet space, sit comfortably, close your eyes, take deep breaths, focus only on the air flowing into your nose, down into your lungs, and back out again.
- Hop on one leg and count to 10, then the other and count to 10
- Do 35 Jumping Jacks
- Do 25 sit-ups or hula hoop for 35 seconds in one direction and 35 seconds in the other direction
- Do arm circles 20 forward, 20 backward, big or small.
- Eat at least two whole pieces of fruit
- Eat at least **two** cups of vegetables
- 1st goal:
- 2nd goal:
- Something I am thankful for today:
- Something I like about myself:
- Something nice I did for someone else today:

- Notes:

# Day Forty

## Goals

- Drink 6-8 glasses of water (no flavor added, just WATER)
- Go for a walk, jog or march in place for at least 15 minutes
- Shut off all electronics for 7 minutes, go to a quiet space, sit comfortably, close your eyes, take deep breaths, focus only on the air flowing into your nose, down into your lungs, and back out again.
- Hop on one leg and count to 10, then the other and count to 10
- Do 35 Jumping Jacks
- Do **30** sit-ups or hula hoop for **40** seconds in one direction and **40** seconds in the other direction
- Do arm circles 20 forward, 20 backward, big or small.
- Eat at least two whole pieces of fruit
- Eat at least two cups of vegetables
- 1st goal:
- 2nd goal:
- Something I am thankful for today:
- Something I like about myself:
- Something nice I did for someone else today:

- Notes:

# Day Forty-One

## Goals

- Drink 6-8 glasses of water (no flavor added, just WATER)
- Go for a walk, jog or march in place for at least 15 minutes
- Shut off all electronics for 7 minutes, go to a quiet space, sit comfortably, close your eyes, take deep breaths, focus only on the air flowing into your nose, down into your lungs, and back out again.
- Hop on one leg and count to 10, then the other and count to 10
- Do 35 Jumping Jacks
- Do 30 sit-ups or hula hoop for 40 seconds in one direction and 40 seconds in the other direction
- Do arm circles 20 forward, 20 backward, big or small.
- Eat at least two whole pieces of fruit
- Eat at least two cups of vegetables
- 1st goal:
- 2nd goal:
- Something I am thankful for today:
- Something I like about myself:
- Something nice I did for someone else today:

- Notes:

# Day Forty-Two

## Goals

- Drink 6-8 glasses of water (no flavor added, just WATER)
- Go for a walk, jog or march in place for at least 15 minutes
- Shut off all electronics for **8** minutes, go to a quiet space, sit comfortably, close your eyes, take deep breaths, focus only on the air flowing into your nose, down into your lungs, and back out again.
- Hop on one leg and count to 10, then the other and count to 10
- Do 35 Jumping Jacks
- Do 30 sit-ups or hula hoop for 40 seconds in one direction and 40 seconds in the other direction
- Do arm circles **25** forward, **25** backward, big or small.
- Eat at least two whole pieces of fruit
- Eat at least two cups of vegetables
- 1st goal:
- 2nd goal:
- Something I am thankful for today:
- Something I like about myself:
- Something nice I did for someone else today:

- Notes:

# Day Forty-Three

## Goals

- Drink 6-8 glasses of water (no flavor added, just WATER)
- Go for a walk, jog or march in place for at least **17** minutes
- Shut off all electronics for 8 minutes, go to a quiet space, sit comfortably, close your eyes, take deep breaths, focus only on the air flowing into your nose, down into your lungs, and back out again.
- Hop on one leg and count to 10, then the other and count to 10
- Do 35 Jumping Jacks
- Do 30 sit-ups or hula hoop for 40 seconds in one direction and 40 seconds in the other direction
- Do arm circles 25 forward, 25 backward, big or small.
- Eat at least two whole pieces of fruit
- Eat at least two cups of vegetables
- 1st goal:
- 2nd goal:
- Something I am thankful for today:
- Something I like about myself:
- Something nice I did for someone else today:

- Notes:

# Day Forty-Four

## Goals

- Drink 6-8 glasses of water (no flavor added, just WATER)
- Go for a walk, jog or march in place for at least 17 minutes
- Shut off all electronics for 8 minutes, go to a quiet space, sit comfortably, close your eyes, take deep breaths, focus only on the air flowing into your nose, down into your lungs, and back out again.
- Hop on one leg and count to 15, then the other and count to 15
- Do 35 Jumping Jacks
- Do 30 sit-ups or hula hoop for 40 seconds in one direction and 40 seconds in the other direction
- Do arm circles 25 forward, 25 backward, big or small.
- Eat at least two whole pieces of fruit
- Eat at least two cups of vegetables
- 1st goal:
- 2nd goal:
- Something I am thankful for today:
- Something I like about myself:
- Something nice I did for someone else today:

- Notes:

# Day Forty-Five

## Goals

- Drink 6-8 glasses of water (no flavor added, just WATER)
- Go for a walk, jog or march in place for at least 17 minutes
- Shut off all electronics for 8 minutes, go to a quiet space, sit comfortably, close your eyes, take deep breaths, focus only on the air flowing into your nose, down into your lungs, and back out again.
- Hop on one leg and count to 15, then the other and count to 15
- Do **40** Jumping Jacks
- Do 30 sit-ups or hula hoop for 40 seconds in one direction and 40 seconds in the other direction
- Do arm circles 25 forward, 25 backward, big or small.
- Eat at least two whole pieces of fruit
- Eat at least two cups of vegetables
- 1st goal:
- 2nd goal:
- Something I am thankful for today:
- Something I like about myself:
- Something nice I did for someone else today:

- Notes:

# Day Forty-Six

## Goals

- Drink 6-8 glasses of water (no flavor added, just WATER)
- Go for a walk, jog or march in place for at least 17 minutes
- Shut off all electronics for 8 minutes, go to a quiet space, sit comfortably, close your eyes, take deep breaths, focus only on the air flowing into your nose, down into your lungs, and back out again.
- Hop on one leg and count to 15, then the other and count to 15
- Do 40 Jumping Jacks
- Do 30 sit-ups or hula hoop for 40 seconds in one direction and 40 seconds in the other direction
- Do arm circles 25 forward, 25 backward, big or small.
- Eat at least two whole pieces of fruit
- Eat at least **two and a half** cups of vegetables
- 1st goal:
- 2nd goal:
- Something I am thankful for today:
- Something I like about myself:
- Something nice I did for someone else today:

- Notes:

# Day Forty-Seven

## Goals

- Drink 6-8 glasses of water (no flavor added, just WATER)
- Go for a walk, jog or march in place for at least 17 minutes
- Shut off all electronics for 8 minutes, go to a quiet space, sit comfortably, close your eyes, take deep breaths, focus only on the air flowing into your nose, down into your lungs, and back out again.
- Hop on one leg and count to 15, then the other and count to 15
- Do 40 Jumping Jacks
- Do **35** sit-ups or hula hoop for **45** seconds in one direction and **45** seconds in the other direction
- Do arm circles 25 forward, 25 backward, big or small.
- Eat at least two whole pieces of fruit
- Eat at least two and a half cups of vegetables
- 1st goal:
- 2nd goal:
- Something I am thankful for today:
- Something I like about myself:
- Something nice I did for someone else today:

- Notes:

# Day Forty-Eight

## Goals

- Drink 6-8 glasses of water (no flavor added, just WATER)
- Go for a walk, jog or march in place for at least 17 minutes
- Shut off all electronics for 8 minutes, go to a quiet space, sit comfortably, close your eyes, take deep breaths, focus only on the air flowing into your nose, down into your lungs, and back out again.
- Hop on one leg and count to 15, then the other and count to 15
- Do 40 Jumping Jacks
- Do 35 sit-ups or hula hoop for 45 seconds in one direction and 45 seconds in the other direction
- Do arm circles 25 forward, 25 backward, big or small.
- Eat at least two whole pieces of fruit
- Eat at least two and a half cups of vegetables
- 1st goal:
- 2nd goal:
- Something I am thankful for today:
- Something I like about myself:
- Something nice I did for someone else today:

- Notes:

# Day Forty-Nine

## Goals

- Drink 6-8 glasses of water (no flavor added, just WATER)
- Go for a walk, jog or march in place for at least 17 minutes
- Shut off all electronics for **9** minutes, go to a quiet space, sit comfortably, close your eyes, take deep breaths, focus only on the air flowing into your nose, down into your lungs, and back out again.
- Hop on one leg and count to 15, then the other and count to 15
- Do 40 Jumping Jacks
- Do 35 sit-ups or hula hoop for 45 seconds in one direction and 45 seconds in the other direction
- Do arm circles **30** forward, **30** backward, big or small.
- Eat at least two whole pieces of fruit
- Eat at least two and a half cups of vegetables
- 1st goal:
- 2nd goal:
- Something I am thankful for today:
- Something I like about myself:
- Something nice I did for someone else today:

- Notes:

# Day Fifty

## Goals

- Drink 6-8 glasses of water (no flavor added, just WATER)
- Go for a walk, jog or march in place for at least **19** minutes
- Shut off all electronics for 9 minutes, go to a quiet space, sit comfortably, close your eyes, take deep breaths, focus only on the air flowing into your nose, down into your lungs, and back out again.
- Hop on one leg and count to 15, then the other and count to 15
- Do 40 Jumping Jacks
- Do 35 sit-ups or hula hoop for 45 seconds in one direction and 45 seconds in the other direction
- Do arm circles 30 forward, 30 backward, big or small.
- Eat at least two whole pieces of fruit
- Eat at least two and a half cups of vegetables
- 1st goal:
- 2nd goal:
- Something I am thankful for today:
- Something I like about myself:
- Something nice I did for someone else today:

- Notes:

# Day Fifty-One

## Goals

- Drink 6-8 glasses of water (no flavor added, just WATER)
- Go for a walk, jog or march in place for at least 19 minutes
- Shut off all electronics for 9 minutes, go to a quiet space, sit comfortably, close your eyes, take deep breaths, focus only on the air flowing into your nose, down into your lungs, and back out again.
- Hop on one leg and count to **20**, then the other and count to **20**
- Do 40 Jumping Jacks
- Do 35 sit-ups or hula hoop for 45 seconds in one direction and 45 seconds in the other direction
- Do arm circles 30 forward, 30 backward, big or small.
- Eat at least two whole pieces of fruit
- Eat at least two and a half cups of vegetables
- 1st goal:
- 2nd goal:
- Something I am thankful for today:
- Something I like about myself:
- Something nice I did for someone else today:

- Notes:

# Day Fifty-Two

## Goals

- Drink 6-8 glasses of water (no flavor added, just WATER)
- Go for a walk, jog or march in place for at least 19 minutes
- Shut off all electronics for 9 minutes, go to a quiet space, sit comfortably, close your eyes, take deep breaths, focus only on the air flowing into your nose, down into your lungs, and back out again.
- Hop on one leg and count to 20, then the other and count to 20
- Do **45** Jumping Jacks
- Do 35 sit-ups or hula hoop for 45 seconds in one direction and 45 seconds in the other direction
- Do arm circles 30 forward, 30 backward, big or small.
- Eat at least two whole pieces of fruit
- Eat at least two and a half cups of vegetables
- 1st goal:
- 2nd goal:
- Something I am thankful for today:
- Something I like about myself:
- Something nice I did for someone else today:

- Notes:

# Day Fifty-Three

## Goals

- Drink 6-8 glasses of water (no flavor added, just WATER)
- Go for a walk, jog or march in place for at least 19 minutes
- Shut off all electronics for 9 minutes, go to a quiet space, sit comfortably, close your eyes, take deep breaths, focus only on the air flowing into your nose, down into your lungs, and back out again.
- Hop on one leg and count to 20, then the other and count to 20
- Do 45 Jumping Jacks
- Do 35 sit-ups or hula hoop for 45 seconds in one direction and 45 seconds in the other direction
- Do arm circles 30 forward, 30 backward, big or small.
- Eat at least two whole pieces of fruit
- Eat at least two and a half cups of vegetables
- 1st goal:
- 2nd goal:
- Something I am thankful for today:
- Something I like about myself:
- Something nice I did for someone else today:

- Notes:

# Day Fifty-Four

## Goals

- Drink 6-8 glasses of water (no flavor added, just WATER)
- Go for a walk, jog or march in place for at least 19 minutes
- Shut off all electronics for 9 minutes, go to a quiet space, sit comfortably, close your eyes, take deep breaths, focus only on the air flowing into your nose, down into your lungs, and back out again.
- Hop on one leg and count to 20, then the other and count to 20
- Do 45 Jumping Jacks
- Do **40** sit-ups or hula hoop for **50** seconds in one direction and **50** seconds in the other direction
- Do arm circles 30 forward, 30 backward, big or small.
- Eat at least two whole pieces of fruit
- Eat at least two and a half cups of vegetables
- 1st goal:
- 2nd goal:
- Something I am thankful for today:
- Something I like about myself:
- Something nice I did for someone else today:

- Notes:

# Day Fifty-Five

## Goals

- Drink 6-8 glasses of water (no flavor added, just WATER)
- Go for a walk, jog or march in place for at least 19 minutes
- Shut off all electronics for 9 minutes, go to a quiet space, sit comfortably, close your eyes, take deep breaths, focus only on the air flowing into your nose, down into your lungs, and back out again.
- Hop on one leg and count to 20, then the other and count to 20
- Do 45 Jumping Jacks
- Do 40 sit-ups or hula hoop for 50 seconds in one direction and 50 seconds in the other direction
- Do arm circles 30 forward, 30 backward, big or small.
- Eat at least two whole pieces of fruit
- Eat at least two and a half cups of vegetables
- 1st goal:
- 2nd goal:
- Something I am thankful for today:
- Something I like about myself:
- Something nice I did for someone else today:

- Notes:

# Day Fifty-Six

## Goals

- Drink 6-8 glasses of water (no flavor added, just WATER)
- Go for a walk, jog or march in place for at least 19 minutes
- Shut off all electronics for **10** minutes, go to a quiet space, sit comfortably, close your eyes, take deep breaths, focus only on the air flowing into your nose, down into your lungs, and back out again.
- Hop on one leg and count to 20, then the other and count to 20
- Do 45 Jumping Jacks
- Do 40 sit-ups or hula hoop for 50 seconds in one direction and 50 seconds in the other direction
- Do arm circles **20** forward, **20** backward, big **and** small.
- Eat at least two whole pieces of fruit
- Eat at least two and a half cups of vegetables
- 1st goal:
- 2nd goal:
- Something I am thankful for today:
- Something I like about myself:
- Something nice I did for someone else today:

- Notes:

# Day Fifty-Seven

## Goals

• Drink 6-8 glasses of water (no flavor added, just WATER)
• Go for a walk, jog or march in place for at least **21 minutes**
• Shut off all electronics for 10 minutes, go to a quiet space, sit comfortably, close your eyes, take deep breaths, focus only on the air flowing into your nose, down into your lungs, and back out again.
• Hop on one leg and count to 20, then the other and count to 20
• Do 45 Jumping Jacks
• Do 40 sit-ups or hula hoop for 50 seconds in one direction and 50 seconds in the other direction
• Do arm circles 20 forward, 20 backward, big and small.
• Eat at least two whole pieces of fruit
• Eat at least two and a half cups of vegetables
• 1st goal:
• 2nd goal:
• Something I am thankful for today:
• Something I like about myself:
• Something nice I did for someone else today:

• Notes:

# Day Fifty-Eight

## Goals

- Drink 6-8 glasses of water (no flavor added, just WATER)
- Go for a walk, jog or march in place for at least 21 minutes
- Shut off all electronics for 10 minutes, go to a quiet space, sit comfortably, close your eyes, take deep breaths, focus only on the air flowing into your nose, down into your lungs, and back out again.
- Hop on one leg and count to **25**, then the other and count to **25**
- Do 45 Jumping Jacks
- Do 40 sit-ups or hula hoop for 50 seconds in one direction and 50 seconds in the other direction
- Do arm circles 20 forward, 20 backward, big and small.
- Eat at least two whole pieces of fruit
- Eat at least two and a half cups of vegetables
- 1st goal:
- 2nd goal:
- Something I am thankful for today:
- Something I like about myself:
- Something nice I did for someone else today:

- Notes:

# Day Fifty-Nine

## Goals

- Drink 6-8 glasses of water (no flavor added, just WATER)
- Go for a walk, jog or march in place for at least 21 minutes
- Shut off all electronics for 10 minutes, go to a quiet space, sit comfortably, close your eyes, take deep breaths, focus only on the air flowing into your nose, down into your lungs, and back out again.
- Hop on one leg and count to 25, then the other and count to 25
- Do **50** Jumping Jacks
- Do 40 sit-ups or hula hoop for 50 seconds in one direction and 50 seconds in the other direction
- Do arm circles 20 forward, 20 backward, big and small.
- Eat at least two whole pieces of fruit
- Eat at least two and a half cups of vegetables
- 1st goal:
- 2nd goal:
- Something I am thankful for today:
- Something I like about myself:
- Something nice I did for someone else today:

- Notes:

# Day Sixty

## Goals

- Drink 6-8 glasses of water (no flavor added, just WATER)
- Go for a walk, jog or march in place for at least 21 minutes
- Shut off all electronics for 10 minutes, go to a quiet space, sit comfortably, close your eyes, take deep breaths, focus only on the air flowing into your nose, down into your lungs, and back out again.
- Hop on one leg and count to 25, then the other and count to 25
- Do 50 Jumping Jacks
- Do 40 sit-ups or hula hoop for 50 seconds in one direction and 50 seconds in the other direction
- Do arm circles 20 forward, 20 backward, big and small.
- Eat at least two whole pieces of fruit
- Eat at least two and a half cups of vegetables
- 1st goal:
- 2nd goal:
- Something I am thankful for today:
- Something I like about myself:
- Something nice I did for someone else today:

- Notes:

# Day Sixty-One

## Goals

- Drink 6-8 glasses of water (no flavor added, just WATER)
- Go for a walk or march in place for at least 21 minutes
- Shut off all electronics for 10 minutes, go to a quiet space, sit comfortably, close your eyes, take deep breaths, focus only on the air flowing into your nose, down into your lungs, and back out again.
- Hop on one leg and count to 25, then the other and count to 25
- Do 50 Jumping Jacks
- Do 40 sit-ups or hula hoop for 50 seconds in one direction and 50 seconds in the other direction
- Do arm circles 20 forward, 20 backward, big and small.
- **Do 3 push-ups (on your knees or on your toes)**
- Eat at least two whole pieces of fruit
- Eat at least two and a half cups of vegetables
- 1st goal:
- 2nd goal:
- Something I am thankful for today:
- Something I like about myself:
- Something nice I did for someone else today:

- Notes:

# Day Sixty-Two

## Goals

- Drink 6-8 glasses of water (no flavor added, just WATER)
- Go for a walk, jog or march in place for at least 21 minutes
- Shut off all electronics for 10 minutes, go to a quiet space, sit comfortably, close your eyes, take deep breaths, focus only on the air flowing into your nose, down into your lungs, and back out again.
- Hop on one leg and count to 25, then the other and count to 25
- Do 50 Jumping Jacks
- Do **45** sit-ups or hula hoop for **55** seconds in one direction and **55** seconds in the other direction
- Do arm circles 20 forward, 20 backward, big and small.
- Do 3 push-ups
- Eat at least two whole pieces of fruit
- Eat at least two and a half cups of vegetables
- 1st goal:
- 2nd goal:
- Something I am thankful for today:
- Something I like about myself:
- Something nice I did for someone else today:

- Notes:

# Day Sixty-Three

## Goals

- Drink 6-8 glasses of water (no flavor added, just WATER)
- Go for a walk, jog or march in place for at least 21 minutes
- Shut off all electronics for 10 minutes, go to a quiet space, sit comfortably, close your eyes, take deep breaths, focus only on the air flowing into your nose, down into your lungs, and back out again.
- Hop on one leg and count to 25, then the other and count to 25
- Do 50 Jumping Jacks
- Do 45 sit-ups or hula hoop for 55 seconds in one direction and 55 seconds in the other direction
- Do arm circles 20 forward, 20 backward, **small, medium, large**
- Do 3 push-ups
- Eat at least two whole pieces of fruit
- Eat at least two and a half cups of vegetables
- 1st goal: **(change or keep)**
- 2nd goal: **(change or keep)**
- **Time for a new goal: (doesn't have to be health related)**
- Something I am thankful for today:
- Something I like about myself:
- Something nice I did for someone else today:

- Notes:

# Day Sixty-Four

## Goals

- Drink 6-8 glasses of water (no flavor added, just WATER)
- Go for a walk, jog or march in place for at least **23** minutes
- Shut off all electronics for 10 minutes, go to a quiet space, sit comfortably, close your eyes, take deep breaths, focus only on the air flowing into your nose, down into your lungs, and back out again.
- Hop on one leg and count to 25, then the other and count to 25
- Do 50 Jumping Jacks
- Do 45 sit-ups or hula hoop for 55 seconds in one direction and 55 seconds in the other direction
- Do arm circles 20 forward, 20 backward, small, medium, large
- Do 3 push-ups
- Eat at least two whole pieces of fruit
- Eat at least two and a half cups of vegetables
- 1st goal:
- 2nd goal:
- 3rd goal:
- Something I am thankful for today:
- Something I like about myself:
- Something nice I did for someone else today:

- Notes:

# Day Sixty-Five

## Goals

- Drink 6-8 glasses of water (no flavor added, just WATER)
- Go for a walk, jog or march in place for at least 23 minutes
- Shut off all electronics for 10 minutes, go to a quiet space, sit comfortably, close your eyes, take deep breaths, focus only on the air flowing into your nose, down into your lungs, and back out again.
- Hop on one leg and count to **30**, then the other and count to **30**
- Do 50 Jumping Jacks
- Do 45 sit-ups or hula hoop for 55 seconds in one direction and 55 seconds in the other direction
- Do arm circles 20 forward, 20 backward, small, medium, large
- Do 3 push-ups
- Eat at least two whole pieces of fruit
- Eat at least two and a half cups of vegetables
- 1st goal:
- 2nd goal:
- 3rd goal:
- Something I am thankful for today:
- Something I like about myself:
- Something nice I did for someone else today:

- Notes:

# Day Sixty-Six

## Goals

- Drink 6-8 glasses of water (no flavor added, just WATER)
- Go for a walk, jog or march in place for at least 23 minutes
- Shut off all electronics for 10 minutes, go to a quiet space, sit comfortably, close your eyes, take deep breaths, focus only on the air flowing into your nose, down into your lungs, and back out again.
- Hop on one leg and count to 30, then the other and count to 30
- Do **55 Jumping Jacks**
- Do 45 sit-ups or hula hoop for 55 seconds in one direction and 55 seconds in the other direction
- Do arm circles 20 forward, 20 backward, small, medium, large
- Do 3 push-ups
- Eat at least two whole pieces of fruit
- Eat at least two and a half cups of vegetables
- 1st goal:
- 2nd goal:
- 3rd goal:
- Something I am thankful for today:
- Something I like about myself:
- Something nice I did for someone else today:

- Notes:

# Day Sixty-Seven

## Goals

- Drink 6-8 glasses of water (no flavor added, just WATER)
- Go for a walk, jog or march in place for at least 23 minutes
- Shut off all electronics for 10 minutes, go to a quiet space, sit comfortably, close your eyes, take deep breaths, focus only on the air flowing into your nose, down into your lungs, and back out again.
- Hop on one leg and count to 30, then the other and count to 30
- Do 55 Jumping Jacks
- Do 45 sit-ups or hula hoop for 55 seconds in one direction and 55 seconds in the other direction
- Do arm circles 20 forward, 20 backward, small, medium, large
- Do 3 push-ups
- Eat at least two whole pieces of fruit
- Eat at least two and a half cups of vegetables
- 1st goal:
- 2nd goal:
- 3rd goal:
- Something I am thankful for today:
- Something I like about myself:
- Something nice I did for someone else today:

- Notes:

# Day Sixty-Eight

## Goals

- Drink 6-8 glasses of water (no flavor added, just WATER)
- Go for a walk, jog or march in place for at least 23 minutes
- Shut off all electronics for 10 minutes, go to a quiet space, sit comfortably, close your eyes, take deep breaths, focus only on the air flowing into your nose, down into your lungs, and back out again.
- Hop on one leg and count to 30, then the other and count to 30
- Do 55 Jumping Jacks
- Do 45 sit-ups or hula hoop for 55 seconds in one direction and 55 seconds in the other direction
- Do arm circles 20 forward, 20 backward, small, medium, large
- Do **5** push-ups
- Eat at least two whole pieces of fruit
- Eat at least two and a half cups of vegetables
- 1st goal:
- 2nd goal:
- 3rd goal:
- Something I am thankful for today:
- Something I like about myself:
- Something nice I did for someone else today:

- Notes:

# Day Sixty-Nine

## Goals

- Drink 6-8 glasses of water (no flavor added, just WATER)
- Go for a walk, jog or march in place for at least 23 minutes
- Shut off all electronics for 10 minutes, go to a quiet space, sit comfortably, close your eyes, take deep breaths, focus only on the air flowing into your nose, down into your lungs, and back out again.
- Hop on one leg and count to 30, then the other and count to 30
- Do 55 Jumping Jacks
- Do **50** sit-ups or hula hoop for **60** seconds in one direction and **60** seconds in the other direction
- Do arm circles 20 forward, 20 backward, small, medium, large
- Do 5 push-ups
- Eat at least two whole pieces of fruit
- Eat at least two and a half cups of vegetables
- 1st goal:
- 2nd goal:
- 3rd goal:
- Something I am thankful for today:
- Something I like about myself:
- Something nice I did for someone else today:

- Notes:

# Day Seventy

## Goals

- Drink 6-8 glasses of water (no flavor added, just WATER)
- Go for a walk, jog or march in place for at least 23 minutes
- Shut off all electronics for 10 minutes, go to a quiet space, sit comfortably, close your eyes, take deep breaths, focus only on the air flowing into your nose, down into your lungs, and back out again.
- Hop on one leg and count to 30, then the other and count to 30
- Do 55 Jumping Jacks
- Do 50 sit-ups or hula hoop for 60 seconds in one direction and 60 seconds in the other direction
- Do arm circles 25 forward, 25 backward, small, medium, large
- Do 5 push-ups
- Eat at least two whole pieces of fruit
- Eat at least two and a half cups of vegetables
- 1st goal:
- 2nd goal:
- 3rd goal:
- Something I am thankful for today:
- Something I like about myself:
- Something nice I did for someone else today:

- Notes:

# Day Seventy-One

## Goals

- Drink 6-8 glasses of water (no flavor added, just WATER)
- Go for a walk, jog or march in place for at least **25** minutes
- Shut off all electronics for 10 minutes, go to a quiet space, sit comfortably, close your eyes, take deep breaths, focus only on the air flowing into your nose, down into your lungs, and back out again.
- Hop on one leg and count to 30, then the other and count to 30
- Do 55 Jumping Jacks
- Do 50 sit-ups or hula hoop for 60 seconds in one direction and 60 seconds in the other direction
- Do arm circles 25 forward, 25 backward, small, medium, large
- Do 5 push-ups
- Eat at least two whole pieces of fruit
- Eat at least two and a half cups of vegetables
- 1st goal:
- 2nd goal:
- 3rd goal:
- Something I am thankful for today:
- Something I like about myself:
- Something nice I did for someone else today:

- Notes:

# Day Seventy-Two

## Goals

- Drink 6-8 glasses of water (no flavor added, just WATER)
- Go for a walk, jog or march in place for at least 25 minutes
- Shut off all electronics for 10 minutes, go to a quiet space, sit comfortably, close your eyes, take deep breaths, focus only on the air flowing into your nose, down into your lungs, and back out again.
- Hop on one leg and count to **35**, then the other and count to **35**
- Do 55 Jumping Jacks
- Do 50 sit-ups or hula hoop for 60 seconds in one direction and 60 seconds in the other direction
- Do arm circles 25 forward, 25 backward, small, medium, large
- Do 5 push-ups
- Eat at least two whole pieces of fruit
- Eat at least two and a half cups of vegetables
- 1st goal:
- 2nd goal:
- 3rd goal:
- Something I am thankful for today:
- Something I like about myself:
- Something nice I did for someone else today:

- Notes:

# Day Seventy-Three

## Goals

- Drink 6-8 glasses of water (no flavor added, just WATER)
- Go for a walk, jog or march in place for at least 25 minutes
- Shut off all electronics for 10 minutes, go to a quiet space, sit comfortably, close your eyes, take deep breaths, focus only on the air flowing into your nose, down into your lungs, and back out again.
- Hop on one leg and count to 35, then the other and count to 35
- Do **60** Jumping Jacks
- Do 50 sit-ups or hula hoop for 60 seconds in one direction and 60 seconds in the other direction
- Do arm circles 25 forward, 25 backward, small, medium, large
- Do 5 push-ups
- Eat at least two whole pieces of fruit
- Eat at least two and a half cups of vegetables
- 1st goal:
- 2nd goal:
- 3rd goal:
- Something I am thankful for today:
- Something I like about myself:
- Something nice I did for someone else today:

- Notes:

# Day Seventy-Four

## Goals

- Drink 6-8 glasses of water (no flavor added, just WATER)
- Go for a walk, jog or march in place for at least 25 minutes
- Shut off all electronics for 10 minutes, go to a quiet space, sit comfortably, close your eyes, take deep breaths, focus only on the air flowing into your nose, down into your lungs, and back out again.
- Hop on one leg and count to 35, then the other and count to 35
- Do 60 Jumping Jacks
- Do 50 sit-ups or hula hoop for 60 seconds in one direction and 60 seconds in the other direction
- Do arm circles 25 forward, 25 backward, small, medium, large
- Do 5 push-ups
- Eat at least two whole pieces of fruit
- Eat at least two and a half cups of vegetables
- 1st goal:
- 2nd goal:
- 3rd goal:
- Something I am thankful for today:
- Something I like about myself:
- Something nice I did for someone else today:

- Notes:

# Day Seventy-Five

## Goals

- Drink 6-8 glasses of water (no flavor added, just WATER)
- Go for a walk, jog or march in place for at least 25 minutes
- Shut off all electronics for 10 minutes, go to a quiet space, sit comfortably, close your eyes, take deep breaths, focus only on the air flowing into your nose, down into your lungs, and back out again.
- Hop on one leg and count to 35, then the other and count to 35
- Do 60 Jumping Jacks
- Do 50 sit-ups or hula hoop for 60 seconds in one direction and 60 seconds in the other direction
- Do arm circles 25 forward, 25 backward, small, medium, large
- Do **7** push-ups
- Eat at least two whole pieces of fruit
- Eat at least two and a half cups of vegetables
- 1st goal:
- 2nd goal:
- 3rd goal:
- Something I am thankful for today:
- Something I like about myself:
- Something nice I did for someone else today:

- Notes:

# Day Seventy-Six

## Goals

- Drink 6-8 glasses of water (no flavor added, just WATER)
- Go for a walk, jog or march in place for at least 25 minutes
- Shut off all electronics for 10 minutes, go to a quiet space, sit comfortably, close your eyes, take deep breaths, focus only on the air flowing into your nose, down into your lungs, and back out again.
- Hop on one leg and count to 35, then the other and count to 35
- Do 60 Jumping Jacks
- Do 50 sit-ups or hula hoop for 60 seconds in one direction and 60 seconds in the other direction
- Do arm circles 25 forward, 25 backward, small, medium, large
- Do 7 push-ups
- Eat at least two whole pieces of fruit
- Eat at least two and a half cups of vegetables
- 1st goal:
- 2nd goal:
- 3rd goal:
- Something I am thankful for today:
- Something I like about myself:
- Something nice I did for someone else today:

- Notes:

# Day Seventy-Seven

## Goals

- Drink 6-8 glasses of water (no flavor added, just WATER)
- Go for a walk, jog or march in place for at least 25 minutes
- Shut off all electronics for 10 minutes, go to a quiet space, sit comfortably, close your eyes, take deep breaths, focus only on the air flowing into your nose, down into your lungs, and back out again.
- Hop on one leg and count to 35, then the other and count to 35
- Do 60 Jumping Jacks
- Do 50 sit-ups or hula hoop for 60 seconds in one direction and 60 seconds in the other direction
- Do arm circles **30** forward, **30** backward, small, medium, large
- Do 7 push-ups
- Eat at least two whole pieces of fruit
- Eat at least two and a half cups of vegetables
- 1st goal:
- 2nd goal:
- 3rd goal:
- Something I am thankful for today:
- Something I like about myself:
- Something nice I did for someone else today:

- Notes:

# Day Seventy-Eight

## Goals

- Drink 6-8 glasses of water (no flavor added, just WATER)
- Go for a walk, jog or march in place for at least **27** minutes
- Shut off all electronics for 10 minutes, go to a quiet space, sit comfortably, close your eyes, take deep breaths, focus only on the air flowing into your nose, down into your lungs, and back out again.
- Hop on one leg and count to 35, then the other and count to 35
- Do 60 Jumping Jacks
- Do 50 sit-ups or hula hoop for 60 seconds in one direction and 60 seconds in the other direction
- Do arm circles 30 forward, 30 backward, small, medium, large
- Do 7 push-ups
- Eat at least two whole pieces of fruit
- Eat at least two and a half cups of vegetables
- 1st goal:
- 2nd goal:
- 3rd goal:
- Something I am thankful for today:
- Something I like about myself:
- Something nice I did for someone else today:

- Notes:

# Day Seventy-Nine

## Goals

- Drink 6-8 glasses of water (no flavor added, just WATER)
- Go for a walk, jog or march in place for at least 27 minutes
- Shut off all electronics for 10 minutes, go to a quiet space, sit comfortably, close your eyes, take deep breaths, focus only on the air flowing into your nose, down into your lungs, and back out again.
- Hop on one leg and count to **40**, then the other and count to **40**
- Do 60 Jumping Jacks
- Do 50 sit-ups or hula hoop for 60 seconds in one direction and 60 seconds in the other direction
- Do arm circles 30 forward, 30 backward, small, medium, large
- Do 7 push-ups
- Eat at least two whole pieces of fruit
- Eat at least two and a half cups of vegetables
- 1st goal:
- 2nd goal:
- 3rd goal:
- Something I am thankful for today:
- Something I like about myself:
- Something nice I did for someone else today:

- Notes:

# Day Eighty

## Goals

- Drink 6-8 glasses of water (no flavor added, just WATER)
- Go for a walk, jog or march in place for at least 27 minutes
- Shut off all electronics for 10 minutes, go to a quiet space, sit comfortably, close your eyes, take deep breaths, focus only on the air flowing into your nose, down into your lungs, and back out again.
- Hop on one leg and count to 40, then the other and count to 40
- Do 60 Jumping Jacks
- Do 50 sit-ups or hula hoop for 60 seconds in one direction and 60 seconds in the other direction
- Do arm circles 30 forward, 30 backward, small, medium, large
- Do 7 push-ups
- Eat at least two whole pieces of fruit
- Eat at least two and a half cups of vegetables
- 1st goal:
- 2nd goal:
- 3rd goal:
- Something I am thankful for today:
- Something I like about myself:
- Something nice I did for someone else today:

- Notes:

# Day Eighty-One

## Goals

- Drink 6-8 glasses of water (no flavor added, just WATER)
- Go for a walk, jog or march in place for at least 27 minutes
- Shut off all electronics for 10 minutes, go to a quiet space, sit comfortably, close your eyes, take deep breaths, focus only on the air flowing into your nose, down into your lungs, and back out again.
- Hop on one leg and count to 40, then the other and count to 40
- Do 60 Jumping Jacks
- Do 50 sit-ups or hula hoop for 60 seconds in one direction and 60 seconds in the other direction
- Do arm circles 30 forward, 30 backward, small, medium, large
- Do 7 push-ups
- Eat at least two whole pieces of fruit
- Eat at least two and a half cups of vegetables
- 1st goal:
- 2nd goal:
- 3rd goal:
- Something I am thankful for today:
- Something I like about myself:
- Something nice I did for someone else today:

- Notes:

# Day Eighty-Two

## Goals

- Drink 6-8 glasses of water (no flavor added, just WATER)
- Go for a walk, jog or march in place for at least 27 minutes
- Shut off all electronics for 10 minutes, go to a quiet space, sit comfortably, close your eyes, take deep breaths, focus only on the air flowing into your nose, down into your lungs, and back out again.
- Hop on one leg and count to 40, then the other and count to 40
- Do 60 Jumping Jacks
- Do 50 sit-ups or hula hoop for 60 seconds in one direction and 60 seconds in the other direction
- Do arm circles 30 forward, 30 backward, small, medium, large
- Do **9** push-ups
- Eat at least two whole pieces of fruit
- Eat at least two and a half cups of vegetables
- 1st goal:
- 2nd goal:
- 3rd goal:
- Something I am thankful for today:
- Something I like about myself:
- Something nice I did for someone else today:

- Notes:

# Day Eighty-Three

## Goals

- Drink 6-8 glasses of water (no flavor added, just WATER)
- Go for a walk, jog or march in place for at least 27 minutes
- Shut off all electronics for 10 minutes, go to a quiet space, sit comfortably, close your eyes, take deep breaths, focus only on the air flowing into your nose, down into your lungs, and back out again.
- Hop on one leg and count to 40, then the other and count to 40
- Do 60 Jumping Jacks
- Do 50 sit-ups or hula hoop for 60 seconds in one direction and 60 seconds in the other direction
- Do arm circles 30 forward, 30 backward, small, medium, large
- Do 9 push-ups
- Eat at least two whole pieces of fruit
- Eat at least two and a half cups of vegetables
- 1st goal:
- 2nd goal:
- 3rd goal:
- Something I am thankful for today:
- Something I like about myself:
- Something nice I did for someone else today:

- Notes:

# Day Eighty-Four

## Goals

- Drink 6-8 glasses of water (no flavor added, just WATER)
- Go for a walk, jog or march in place for at least 27 minutes
- Shut off all electronics for 10 minutes, go to a quiet space, sit comfortably, close your eyes, take deep breaths, focus only on the air flowing into your nose, down into your lungs, and back out again.
- Hop on one leg and count to 40, then the other and count to 40
- Do 60 Jumping Jacks
- Do 50 sit-ups or hula hoop for 60 seconds in one direction and 60 seconds in the other direction
- Do arm circles 30 forward, 30 backward, small, medium, large
- Do 9 push-ups
- Eat at least two whole pieces of fruit
- Eat at least two and a half cups of vegetables
- 1st goal:
- 2nd goal:
- 3rd goal:
- Something I am thankful for today:
- Something I like about myself:
- Something nice I did for someone else today:

- Notes:

# Day Eighty-Five

## Goals

- Drink 6-8 glasses of water (no flavor added, just WATER)
- Go for a walk, jog or march in place for at least 27 minutes
- Shut off all electronics for 10 minutes, go to a quiet space, sit comfortably, close your eyes, take deep breaths, focus only on the air flowing into your nose, down into your lungs, and back out again.
- Hop on one leg and count to 40, then the other and count to 40
- Do 60 Jumping Jacks
- Do 50 sit-ups or hula hoop for 60 seconds in one direction and 60 seconds in the other direction
- Do arm circles 30 forward, 30 backward, small, medium, large
- Do 9 push-ups
- Eat at least two whole pieces of fruit
- Eat at least two and a half cups of vegetables
- 1st goal:
- 2nd goal:
- 3rd goal:
- Something I am thankful for today:
- Something I like about myself:
- Something nice I did for someone else today:

- Notes:

# Day Eighty-Six

## Goals

- Drink 6-8 glasses of water (no flavor added, just WATER)
- Go for a walk, jog or march in place for at least **30** minutes
- Shut off all electronics for 10 minutes, go to a quiet space, sit comfortably, close your eyes, take deep breaths, focus only on the air flowing into your nose, down into your lungs, and back out again.
- Hop on one leg and count to **45**, then the other and count to **45**
- Do 60 Jumping Jacks
- Do 50 sit-ups or hula hoop for 60 seconds in one direction and 60 seconds in the other direction
- Do arm circles 30 forward, 30 backward, small, medium, large
- Do 9 push-ups
- Eat at least two whole pieces of fruit
- Eat at least two and a half cups of vegetables
- 1st goal:
- 2nd goal:
- 3rd goal:
- Something I am thankful for today:
- Something I like about myself:
- Something nice I did for someone else today:

- Notes:

# Day Eighty-Seven

## Goals

- Drink 6-8 glasses of water (no flavor added, just WATER)
- Go for a walk, jog or march in place for at least 30 minutes
- Shut off all electronics for 10 minutes, go to a quiet space, sit comfortably, close your eyes, take deep breaths, focus only on the air flowing into your nose, down into your lungs, and back out again.
- Hop on one leg and count to 45, then the other and count to 45
- Do 60 Jumping Jacks
- Do 50 sit-ups or hula hoop for 60 seconds in one direction and 60 seconds in the other direction
- Do arm circles 30 forward, 30 backward, small, medium, large
- Do 9 push-ups
- Eat at least two whole pieces of fruit
- Eat at least two and a half cups of vegetables
- 1st goal:
- 2nd goal:
- 3rd goal:
- Something I am thankful for today:
- Something I like about myself:
- Something nice I did for someone else today:

- Notes:

# Day Eighty-Eight

## Goals

- Drink 6-8 glasses of water (no flavor added, just WATER)
- Go for a walk, jog or march in place for at least 30 minutes
- Shut off all electronics for 10 minutes, go to a quiet space, sit comfortably, close your eyes, take deep breaths, focus only on the air flowing into your nose, down into your lungs, and back out again.
- Hop on one leg and count to 45, then the other and count to 45
- Do 60 Jumping Jacks
- Do 50 sit-ups or hula hoop for 60 seconds in one direction and 60 seconds in the other direction
- Do arm circles 30 forward, 30 backward, small, medium, large
- Do 9 push-ups
- Eat at least two whole pieces of fruit
- Eat at least two and a half cups of vegetables
- 1st goal:
- 2nd goal:
- 3rd goal:
- Something I am thankful for today:
- Something I like about myself:
- Something nice I did for someone else today:

- Notes:

# Day Eighty-Nine

## Goals

- Drink 6-8 glasses of water (no flavor added, just WATER)
- Go for a walk, jog or march in place for at least 30 minutes
- Shut off all electronics for 10 minutes, go to a quiet space, sit comfortably, close your eyes, take deep breaths, focus only on the air flowing into your nose, down into your lungs, and back out again.
- Hop on one leg and count to 45, then the other and count to 45
- Do 60 Jumping Jacks
- Do 50 sit-ups or hula hoop for 60 seconds in one direction and 60 seconds in the other direction
- Do arm circles 30 forward, 30 backward, small, medium, large
- Do 10 push-ups
- Eat at least two whole pieces of fruit
- Eat at least two and a half cups of vegetables
- 1st goal:
- 2nd goal:
- 3rd goal:
- Something I am thankful for today:
- Something I like about myself:
- Something nice I did for someone else today:

- Notes:

# Day Ninety

## Goals

- Drink 6-8 glasses of water (no flavor added, just WATER)
- Go for a walk, jog or march in place for at least 30 minutes
- Shut off all electronics for 10 minutes, go to a quiet space, sit comfortably, close your eyes, take deep breaths, focus only on the air flowing into your nose, down into your lungs, and back out again.
- Hop on one leg and count to 45, then the other and count to 45
- Do 60 Jumping Jacks
- Do 50 sit-ups or hula hoop for 60 seconds in one direction and 60 seconds in the other direction
- Do arm circles 30 forward, 30 backward, small, medium, large
- Do 10 push-ups
- Eat at least two whole pieces of fruit
- Eat at least two and a half cups of vegetables
- 1st goal:
- 2nd goal:
- 3rd goal:
- Something I am thankful for today:
- Something I like about myself:
- Something nice I did for someone else today:

- Notes:

# Every Day From Now On

## Goals

- Drink **at least** 6-8 glasses of water (no flavor added, just WATER)
- Go for a walk or jog, or march in place for **at least** 30 minutes
- Shut off all electronics for **at least** 10 minutes, go to a quiet space, sit comfortably, close your eyes, take deep breaths, focus only on the air flowing into your nose, down into your lungs, and back out again.
- Hop on one leg and count to **at least** 45, then the other and count to **at least** 45
- Do **at least** 60 Jumping Jacks
- Do **at least** 50 sit-ups or hula hoop for **at least** 60 seconds in one direction and 60 seconds in the other direction
- Do **at least** 30 arm circles forward, and **at least** 30 backward, small, medium, and large
- Do **at least** 10 push-ups
- Eat **at least** two whole pieces of fruit
- Eat **at least** two and a half cups of vegetables

Continue to work on your own personal goals and create new ones
- 1st goal:
- 2nd goal:
- 3rd goal:

Continue to write down

- Something I am thankful for today:
- Something I like about myself:
- Something nice I did for someone else today:


- Notes:

www.ingramcontent.com/pod-product-compliance
Lightning Source LLC
Chambersburg PA
CBHW050504290526
45786CB00006B/2426